DARING DAMES

A 5-Step Guide to Wellness

Jacqueline Gikow

Audacious Living NYC™

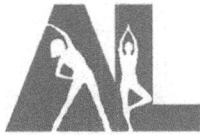

Concept ©2021 Jacqueline Gikow, LLC
Cover copyright ©2021 by Jacqueline Gikow, LLC
Photographs ©2021 Jacqueline Gikow, LLC

Photography by Jacqueline Gikow
Cover design by Jacqueline Gikow
Library of Congress Control Number: 2018675309

Disclaimer: The information in this book supplements, and does not replace, fitness training with a qualified professional. Please consult your personal physician or healthcare specialist before beginning any exercise program.

The publisher and the author make no claims or guarantees about the success you may attain by following these exercises. The author is not a licensed healthcare care provider and has no expertise in diagnosing, examining, or treating medical conditions of any kind, or in determining the effect of any specific exercise on a medical condition.

Every exercise program involving equipment, balance, and movement factors, contains inherent physical risk. If you take part in these exercises, you assume all risk of injury to yourself. You also agree to release and discharge the publisher and the author from any and all claims or causes of action, known or unknown, arising out of the contents of this book. The use of this book implies your acceptance of this disclaimer.

Before practicing the exercises described in this book, be sure your equipment is well maintained. Do not take risks beyond your level of experience, aptitude, training, and comfort level.

DARING DAMES

A 5-Step Guide to Wellness

Table of Contents

Daring Days: Introduction
Chapter 1. Step 1: Get Active — Get Healthy
Chapter 2. Step 2: Manage Your Weight — Eating Well
Chapter 3. Step 3: Build Balance and Flexibility
Chapter 4. Step 4: Mood Modifiers — Choose to be Happier
Chapter 5. Step 5: Habit and Rituals — Find Magic in the Mundane Chapter
Chapter 6. Maintenance and Beyond

Introduction
Daring Dames: A 5-Step Guide to Wellness

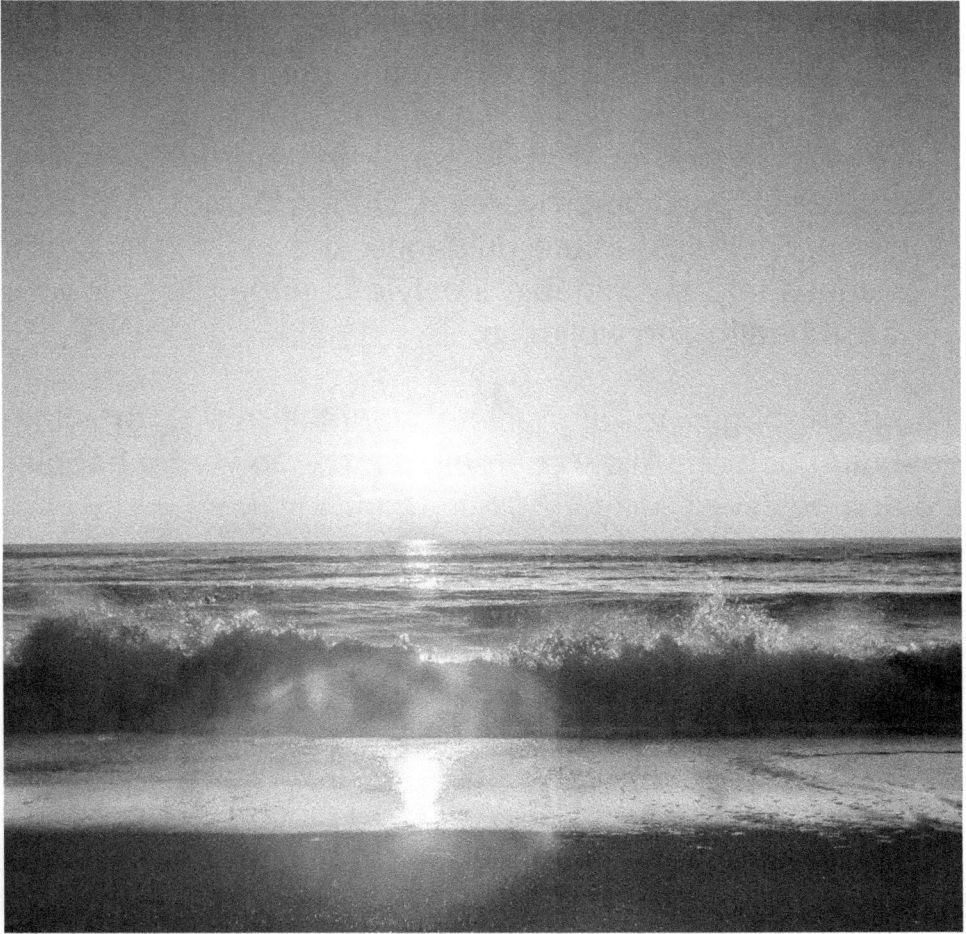

"They always say time changes things, but you actually have to change them yourself."
— Andy Warhol, The Philosophy of Andy Warhol

Daring Dames, A 5-Step Guide to Wellness, can help you:

- Get more active
- Increase your happiness level.
- Get off the diet merry-go-round
- Discover how to have more energy
- Learn how to use small steps to change your habits

Discover a higher level of personal health and wellbeing. With small steps for improvement, Daring Dames, A 5-Step Guide to Wellness, offers guidance and tools. Transform awareness into sustainable lifestyle change. Renew your sense of health and wellness.

You can begin to appreciate yourself as a growing, changing person. Allow yourself to move toward a happier life and positive health.

Health vs. Wellness
The term "health" is mistaken for "wellness." Many people continue to interchange these two words. But health and wellness are not synonyms. Health refers to a physical body being free from diseases. Wellness is balance. It includes our physical, social, spiritual, emotional, intellectual, environmental, and occupational well-being.

Health is someone who wants to lose weight and lower their blood pressure. Once he does reach that goal, he considers himself healthy. Health is a goal to achieve.

Wellness expands our idea of health beyond the simple presence or absence of disease. Wellness is a dynamic concept that continues throughout a lifetime.

Wellness refers to optimal health and vitality — to living life to its fullest. Wellness is a way of living. We have to exert extra effort to experience wellness. We are, thus, asked to take some kind of action.

Health is a state of being. Wellness is about striving for your best balance of all the dimensions above. Wellness is a continuum.

Behaviors That Contribute to Wellness
Good choices and healthy behaviors maximize our quality of life. They help people avoid disease, and remain strong and fit.

Our body works best when it is active. It adapts to most levels of activity and exertion. Physical fitness allows our body to adapt to the demands and stress of physical effort.

Unfortunately, a sedentary lifestyle is common among Americans today. Almost 40% of adult Americans get no leisure-time activity at all.

Physical activity provides physical and mental benefits. The results are immediate as well as long-term. Being fit makes it easier to do everyday tasks and provides strength for emergencies. It helps us look and feel well. Longer term, being fit offers protection against chronic diseases. It lowers the risk of early death.

Active people are less likely to develop or die from many chronic ailments. And they may avoid many problems associated with aging.

Behavior Change

Consider the various behaviors that contribute to wellness. You may make a mental comparison with your own behaviors. Moving towards wellness means cultivating healthy behaviors and ending unhealthy ones.

Changing an unhealthy habit may be harder than it looks. When you embark on a behavior change plan, it may seem like too much work at first. But as you make progress, you gain confidence in your ability to take charge of your life. You will also experience the benefits of energy, vitality, and a higher quality of life.

Be S.M.A.R.T. About Setting Goals

Most of us fail at changing a behavior, not because of a lack of ability. We fail because we never organize our goals. Setting S.M.A.R.T. goals is the first step to make your goal a reality. Smart goals are Specific, Measurable, Achievable, Realistic and Timely.

If your goals are too challenging, you will have trouble making progress and will be more likely to give up. But, if you set goals you can live with, it will be easier to stick with your behavior change plan and be successful.

- ***Specific.*** Avoid vague goals like "get more sleep" Instead, state your objectives in specific terms, such as "turn off the TV an hour before I go to sleep."
- ***Measurable.*** Recognize that your progress will be easier to track if your goals are quantifiable, so give your goal a number. You might measure your goal in terms of time (such as "walk briskly for 20 minutes a day"), distance ("run 2 miles, 3 days per week"), or some other amount ("drink 2 glasses of water when I wake up").
- ***Attainable.*** When you identify goals that are important to you, you can figure out ways to make them come true. You will develop the attitudes, abilities and skills to reach them.
- ***Realistic.*** Your goal is probably realistic if you truly believe that it can be accomplished. A way to know if your goal is realistic is to determine if you have accomplished anything similar in the past or ask yourself what conditions would have to exist to accomplish your goal.
- ***Time-frame specific.*** Give yourself a reasonable amount of time to reach your goal, state the time frame in your behavior change plan, and set your agenda to meet the goal within a given time frame.

Living a healthy lifestyle varies and will be different for each person. It's in our best interest to do things to help ourselves, but that's easier said than done. Most of us are unsuccessful doing helpful things on a global basis. But we can all do small things throughout the day that will help us. Attitude, behavior and lifestyle changes can promote physical, mental/emotional and spiritual health. Maintaining is possible with well-balanced stages of life-wellness. That's why my 5-step guide is a good start.

To achieve wellness, we must balance three core aspects of our life: **mind**, **body**, and **spirit**. The results will be a feeling of wellbeing.

Start by developing a healthy core-level of wellness. Then you can include other ingredients to achieve a high level of well-being.

Wellness is about striving for balance and harmony between each aspect of life-wellness. An imbalance in one has a direct and negative impact on the others. Each part of life-wellness affects the others. So, apply time, effort and care into each. That will encourage the best, well-rounded, well-balanced results. Getting to a healthy state of life-wellness is active and ongoing. It's a dynamic process of awareness, choice, and balance throughout your life.

The Meaning of a Healthy Lifestyle
We want to have a healthy lifestyle, but what does it mean, and how does one go about achieving and maintaining it? Each person must take the time to answer it for himself or herself. It will be different for each of us. And it depends on our situation, attitude, and perception.

Living life to the fullest is about making the most out of our life, situation, and world. It won't help to compare ourselves to a rock star, a movie star, or anyone else for that matter. We are each unique. We have to make the most with what we have and do whatever we can. That's how we improve and evolve as a well-balanced, well-rounded and loving person.

A well-balanced lifestyle is a lifelong effort. It includes striving towards achieving physical, mental, emotional and spiritual health. Behavioral changes are challenging, but achievable with persistence, determination, and the right techniques.

It is really about applying what you learn in an effort to maintain balance while creating healthy ways to improve in all the areas of wellness and lifestyle. Even making small and positive changes in your attitude and behavior can snowball into big, positive results that can improve your lifestyle and contributions to others and the world around you.

Where to start?
Are you excited about creating change to live a healthier, fulfilling lifestyle?

Start by doing one or more of the steps introduced in this book. Make a few changes in each, and you'll plant seeds that can grow and develop into meaningful results.

Make Healthy Decisions

You can make conscious decisions to take positive actions throughout each day. Begin by turning small decisions into actions. Each decision and actions creates positive changes. They add up to results that improve the quality of your day and your lifestyle. While not always obvious, many decisions and actions create long-term benefits. Each one you make adds one drop into a bucket. Taking one step at a time, or laying down one brick at a time to create a wall, helps you build your dream castle. You can be the architect and builder of your life.

It may help to keep a journal. You can note your current situation, state your goals, and track your progress in each area. Journaling is a great tool. The process of writing something down often reinforces your commitment.

Here are five questions that you can ask yourself for each wellness area described in Daring Dames, A 5-Step Guide to Wellness.

Define it: When it comes to your health and wellness, what do you wish were true? Discover your strengths: What conditions would allow you to generate change?

Dream it: What would be your wildest positive solution to achieving wellness?

Design it: What can you commit to for each day make the changes you want?

Your destiny: What would you like to happen?

In A 5-Step Guide to Wellness, you can apply the above questions to each of the following steps:

Chapter 1. Step 1: Get Active — Get Healthy

The first step to wellness is a call to action. I know getting healthy isn't easy! But start now and you'll notice a difference right away. Become fit and you improve your endurance, flexibility and strength.

Chapter 2. Step 2: Manage Your Weight by Eating Well

Oh yeah, your food. Whether we're happy with our weight or not food is always on our minds. Enjoying what we eat is part of what will keep us motivated. We won't get there by beating ourselves up every time we get off track. We get there by being kind to ourselves, having fun and learning along the way.

Chapter 3. Step 3: Build Balance and Flexibility

falls each year. They may suffer moderate to severe injuries, or increase their risk of early death. Taking control of your health to lower your risk of falling. Improve your balance, which tends to decline as we get older.

Chapter 4. Step 4: Mood Modifiers — Choose to be Happier

Choose to be happier means to make a conscious choice to boost your level of happiness. Research reports that we are happier as we get older. But many people don't realize that happiness is a choice. Once you decide to be happier, you can choose strategies for achieving happiness.

Chapter 5. Step 5: Habit and Rituals — Finding Magic in the Mundane

The last step may be the key to achieving the first four. Think about the insignificant decisions you make each day that you take for granted. What if small tweaks to your decisions and actions enhances your life?

Chapter 1
Step 1: Get Active — Get Healthy

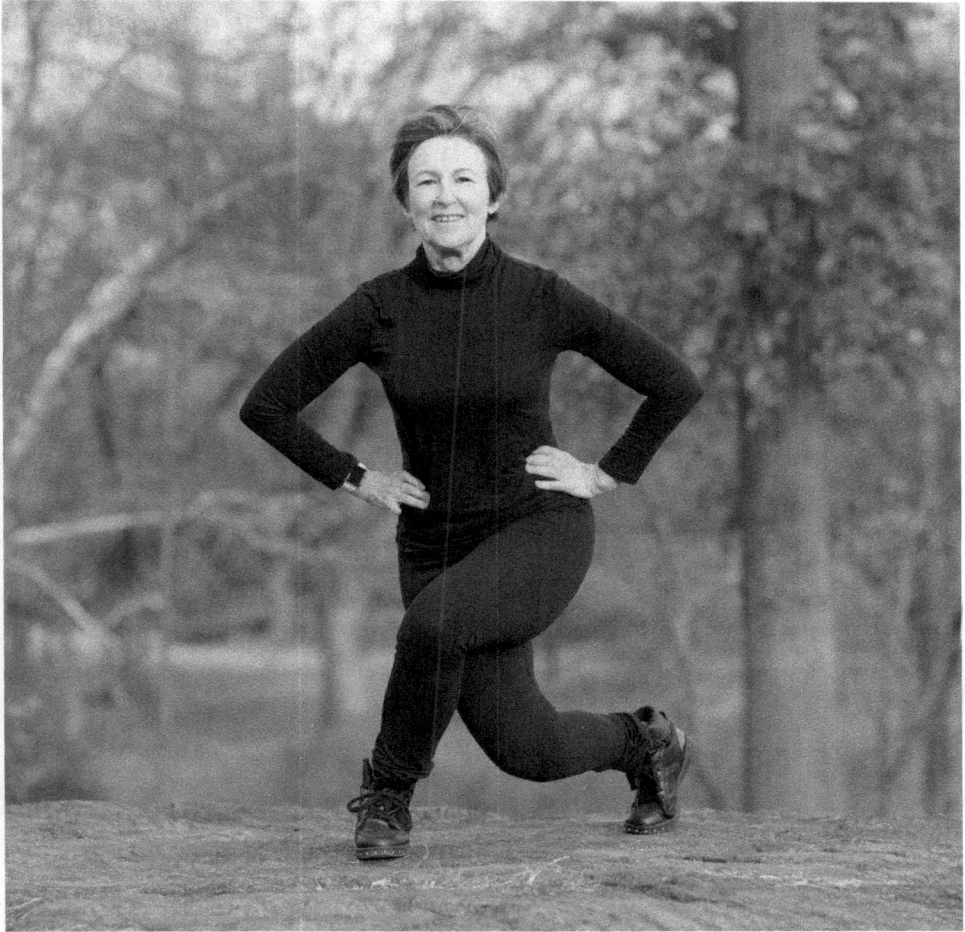

Physical activity is an essential component of a healthy lifestyle. Combined with healthy eating, it can help prevent a range of chronic diseases. Physical activity helps build muscle and lowers fat. It also promotes strong bone, muscles, and joints. All the activities we do all day that involve movement are examples of physical activity.

Physical fitness includes cardiorespiratory endurance. It also includes muscle endurance and strength. Flexibility, balance, agility and coordination are more components of physical fitness. We may reach some health benefits only with strenuous physical activity. Improvement in cardiovascular fitness is one example. Jogging or running has more cardiovascular benefit than slow walking, for instance. Enhanced fitness depends on how much, and for how long, you continue the activity.

So, get active and get healthy for:

A SENSE OF WELL-BEING
Being in good shape can increase your energy, and reduce anxiety and depression. Being active improves your self-esteem and manages your stress.

STRONG BONES
Exercise, foods rich in calcium, is necessary to build strong, healthy bones. Exercising can slow the bone loss associated with getting older.

LOOKING AND FEELING BETTER
You look and feel better when you're in shape and eating right. Being active helps you build muscles and improve your posture. Moving more and eating healthy are important to maintaining a healthy weight.

Getting healthy isn't easy — I know! But start now and you'll notice a difference right away, in your body and your mind. Move more and make healthy eating choices, to improve endurance, flexibility, and strength.

Be S.M.A.R.T. About Setting Goals

Most of us fail at changing a behavior because we don't organize our goals, not because of we lack ability. That's why setting S.M.A.R.T. goals is the first step to make your goal a reality. Smart goals are Specific, Measurable, Achievable, Realistic, and Time-based.

Didn't you read this before? It's still true.

If our goals are too challenging, we have trouble making progress and are more likely to give up. So, set goals you can live with. It is easier be successful with a plan for behavior change.

Setting realistic goals, and sticking to them, is an important part of fitness. Employ the S.M.A.R.T. principle discussed in the first chapter of Daring Dames, A 5-Step Guide to Wellness, and choose goals that are:

S - specific
M - measurable
A - attainable, achievable
R - realistic
T - time-based

Be realistic... Really
Make challenging, but attainable goals. An unreachable goal can be discouraging, as well as disheartening. "I will run a marathon" won't happen immediately, but "I will join a gym this week" may result in success.

Live for the moment.
Think short-term. Set goals that are meaningful and reachable soon. "I will begin a running routine," is an admirable goal. "I will buy new running shoes and plan a one-mile route" is a more workable starting plan.

Keep it simple.
"I'll increase my activity time by 5 minutes each week until I reach 30 minutes a day." Or "I'll drink 8 glasses of water each day this week.

The Basics I — Physical Activity
Physical activity is any movement produced by muscles that requires an energy expenditure. Physical inactivity is the fourth leading risk factor for global mortality. It causes an estimated 3.2 million deaths globally.

Regular moderate intensity physical activity — such as walking, has significant benefits for health. Moderate intensity means breathing harder, but able to speak in full sentences. Moderate intensity activity can reduce the risk depression and of many diseases. And physical activity can help control weight.

Get your heart pumping and your muscles moving. Start an active lifestyle with a goal of moderate activity for 30 minutes a day, at least 5 days a week. Alternatively, you can count your daily activity steps using your phone, smartwatch, or even a pedometer.

Activity is anything that gets your body moving. Start at a comfortable level. Once you get the hang of it, add a little more activity each time. Aim to be active more often. The

Basics II — Physical Fitness
Physical activity includes aerobic and muscle-strengthening activities. If you're just starting, increase your activity over a period of weeks. If you get off track you can always pick up where you dropped off. Your body and mind will start to enjoy physical activity every day.

How hard do you need to push yourself? The right level of effort is: *If you can talk without any trouble at all, you're not working hard enough. If you can't talk at all, it's too hard.*

These are the four phases of physical fitness activity that will ensure you your body is ready to move.

1. Warm Up: Warming up makes our muscles more limber. It decreases our chance of injury during exercise. When we warm up, we increase our blood flow and get our muscles and joints ready to exercise. You'll know you're ready to go when you start to breathe harder.

2. Move: Moving is doing any moderate- to vigorous-intensity activities. Exercise is critical for strong muscles and bones. Muscle strength declines as we get older. But when we move regularly, we can become stronger and leaner than others in our age range (at any age).

3. Cool Down: After exercising, cool down until your breathing is normal and your heartbeat slows down. A cool down involves doing an activity at a slower speed or lower intensity.

4. Stretch: Stretching improves flexibility. After a cool down, stretch the muscles used while you were moving harder. The best approach is to stretch until you feel some tension on the muscle. Flexibility is how much our joint can move between a flexed position and the extended position. Flexible joints can prevent injuries.

Movement Definitions
Aerobic movement is a type of activity that requires oxygen. When exercising, you may notice you're breathing faster and you're getting warmer (you may sweat). Aerobic activities include dancing, swimming, running and bicycling. Aerobic workouts make your heart better at doing its main job — delivering oxygen to all parts of your body.

Muscle-strengthening movement makes your muscles stronger. Muscle-strengthening activities include lifting weights, or using resistance bands. Even using your body weight as a tool can be effective.

Movement Misconceptions
Biological changes, as we grow older, have some physiological effects, but most are side effects of inactivity. We are only somewhat different than our younger counterparts. It isn't possible to reverse biological changes, but we can reduce the impact on our lives.

If we start and keep up an exercise program, we'll see improvements in strength and muscle tone. Bone density, cardiac function, and fat loss also happen. We may not deadlift 400 pounds, but strength gains relative to body weight are possible at any age. Those improvements will show up in the mirror.

Metabolism slowdown: Our metabolism doesn't slow as much we think. Fat gain has more to do with an inactive lifestyle that uses less calories. Losing muscle mass (sarcopenia) makes fat mass seem to increase. What should you do? Get active and modify your diet. Regardless of age, small consistent "wins" result in big changes.

That Persistent Myth
Myths about strength training persist more here than any other area of fitness. For the last time, lifting weights will not turn us into a raging green superhero. Women have 20 to 30 percent less of the hormone testosterone than guys,

so we gain strength without the heft. We'd have to spend 24/7 eating and working out in a specific way in order to bulk up. Our chances of getting scary big? Zilch!

Chapter 2
Step 2: Manage your weight — Eating Well

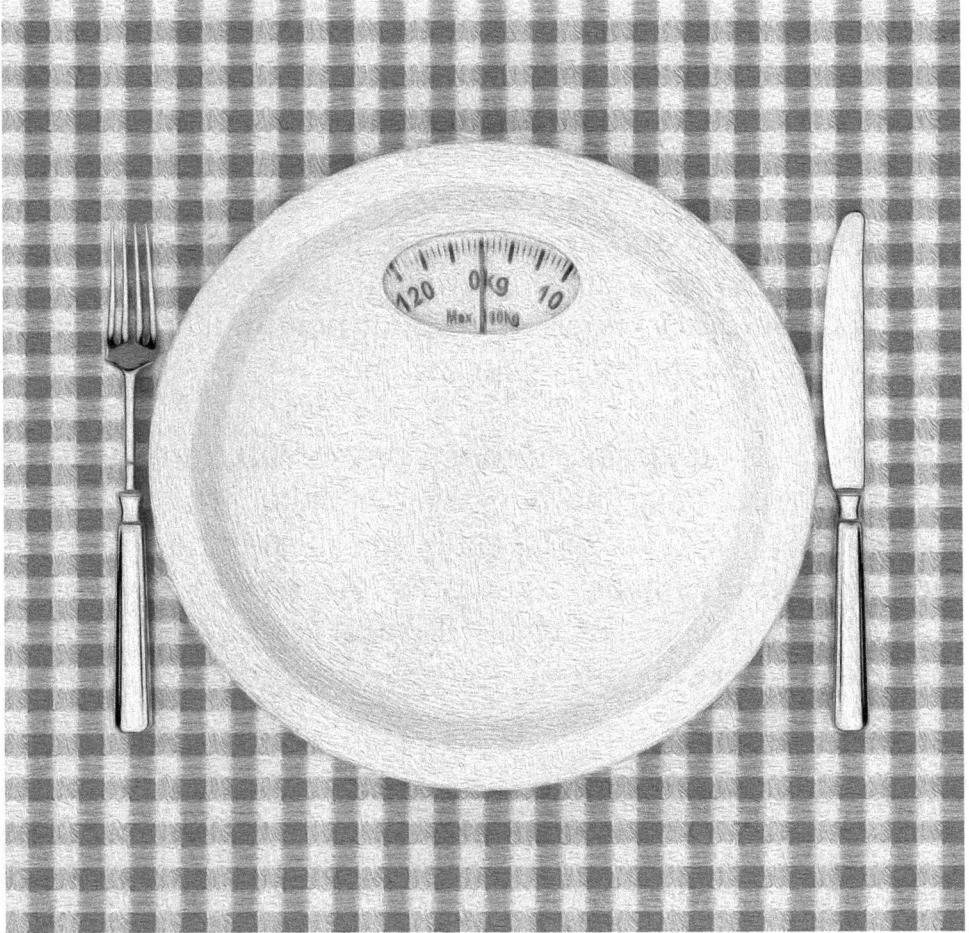

To create a healthy eating practice you can stick with, you have to make a commitment. Losing weight and/or maintaining a healthy weight takes time and effort. It requires you to make some sacrifices. (If it were easy, everyone would be would do it!)

The National Weight Loss Registry reports that people do better when they count calories than when they don't. But that doesn't mean it's for everyone. Counting calories is a tool in our weight loss toolkit and we need to select the tools that are right for us.

Most of us are bad at keeping an honest track of our caloric intake. But being aware caloric content in foods and portions is valuable. A few weeks of tracking can ease you into a portion-controlled approach. Being familiar with calories gives you knowledge about how much you need to eat to lose or maintain your weight.

Calorie counting is simple these days. You don't have to carry a calorie counting book or calculator wherever you go. Apps like *MyFitnessPal* allow you to scan bar codes of food or add eating at restaurants. As always, find what works for you, and stick with it if you enjoy it. Also, *Weight Watchers* (or WW) offers a lifestyle approach to weight management.

Step 1. Set Goals

The first step in establishing a healthy approach to dealing with food, or your weight-loss journey, is to decide what makes sense for you. Assess your eating habits and make a game plan. include long-term and more immediate goals, too.

Step 2. Document Your Progress

Self-awareness begets self-motivation. Keeping track of your behavior motivates you to change because you become more accountable.

Measure Progress with Measurements
Take bi-weekly or monthly measurements at the following spots:
1. Chest - At widest point
2. Waist
3. Hips – About nine inches below hips
4. Shoulders - At widest point
5. Dominant Forearm – Straight elbow,
6. Dominant Upper Arm – Straight elbow
7. Dominant Thigh – Standing
8. Dominant Calf - At widest point

Even if your weight doesn't budge, you'll see the measurements head in the right direction.

Measure Progress with Photos
Taking photos eliminates bias and lets you objectively compare changes.
1. Take 3 photos: front, side, and back.
2. Take photos under the same conditions (lighting, distance from camera, angle, time of day, etc.).
3. Pictures in bathing trunks reveal the most changes.

Step 3. Eat Mindfully and Make it Visible

The key to healthy eating is not to make any food forbidden. Get to know the foods that make your life more comfortable.

Slow Down. A way to make your relationship with food healthier is to take time to eat it. Tracking yourself with a food diary is a powerful tool for managing your weight, eating habits, and relationship to food

Use a notebook to keep a food diary, or use an online tracking system. Eating challenges and exercise goals are easier to meet when tracked. You'll find these benefits of keeping a food diary:

- **Awareness**: You'll be aware not only of how much you eat, but also what you're choosing to put in your mouth. Track everything, from beverages to that handful of grapes.
- **Accountability**: You'll be able to pinpoint when you seem to overeat, and which foods trigger a need to eat more. You'll see the three days you didn't go to the gym during the week. Your journal helps you stay on track.
- **Motivation**: When you feel like you aren't seeing new results fast enough, flip back to the beginning pages of your journal. You'll see you have improved at your own pace. And it will motivate you to stay the course.

- **Celebration**: One of the greatest benefits you can get from a journal is a reason to celebrate. Use the journal to record goals you've achieved. Your journal can be a place to rave about successes.

Step 4. Get Support

Developing a habit of healthy eating is challenging, so don't expect to do it alone. Find a someone you can call on if you need encouragement when you're frustrated. They'll also be companions for celebrating your success.

Weight Loss Stumbling Blocks

When the scale jumps up and down several pounds over the course of a few days, fat isn't the culprit. Something else is going on. Weight can fluctuate 5-10 pounds from the factors below. That's huge. Be patient and amazing results will come.

Muscle Loss can cause weight to drop fast. But faster weight loss isn't always a good thing.

Carbs and Sodium Both of these can cause water retention.

Cortisol, the stress hormone, might be the most frustrating factor. It's hard to measure and can stall your weight for several weeks.

Stress can elevate cortisol. The solution to heightened stress is simple, but not always easy: do something to remove the stress.

Step 5. Change Your Perspective

It's not enough to eat healthy foods and exercise for a few weeks or even months if you want long-term, healthy weight management. Lifestyle changes are necessary as well.

Don't give up, or beat yourself up about a setback. Learn to recognize — and nip a lapse in the bud before it derails your weight management plan.

Chapter 3
Step 3: Build Balance and Flexibility

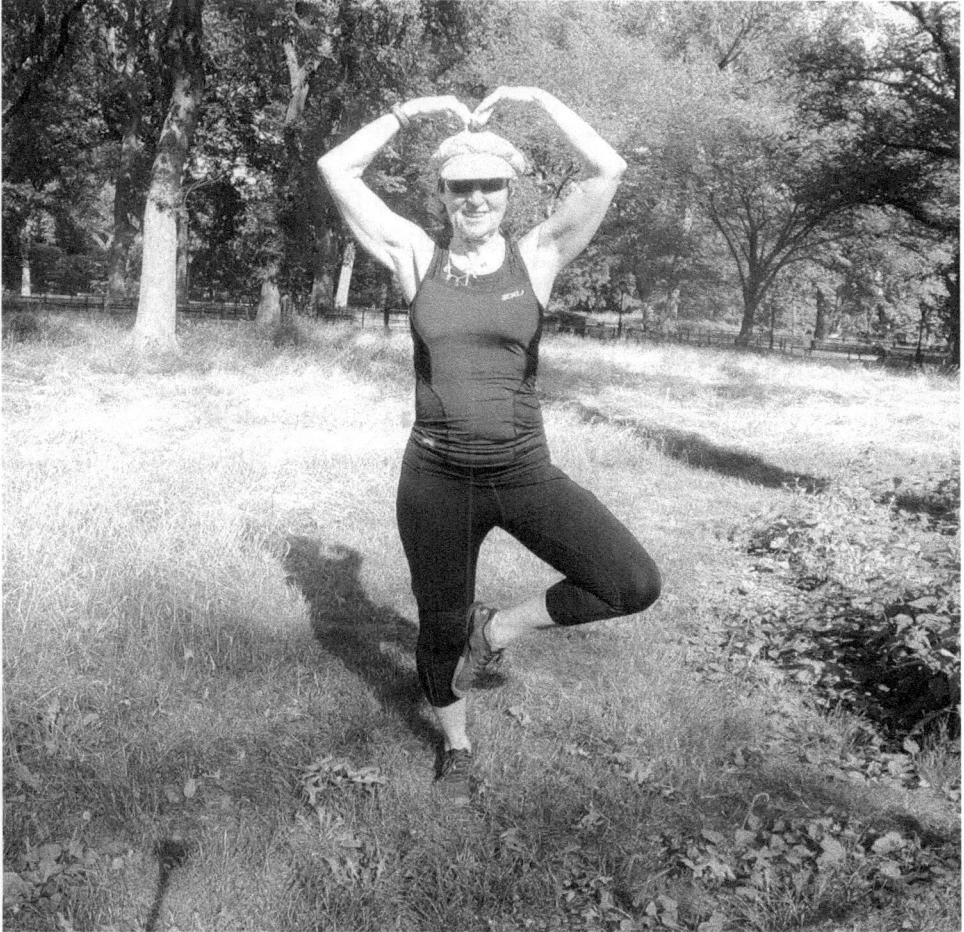

In the United States, one in three adults, aged 65 and older, falls each year. Experiencing moderate to severe injuries increases the risk of early death. Broken bones limit mobility and lead to a downward health spiral. Broken bones and head injuries also knock your confidence. They build a fear of falling, and undermine independence.

But falls are not an inevitable part of aging. You can prevent many falls by following these guidelines:

Move more.
Exercise strengthens weak legs and reduces your chances of falling. Exercise programs such as aquatic fitness safely build strength and improve balance.

Check your medication side effects
Some medicines, or combinations of medicines, have side effects such as dizziness or drowsiness. These can make falling more likely.

Have your eyes checked
Poor vision can make it harder to get around safely. Have your eyes checked every year. And wear glasses or contact lenses with the right prescription.

Improve Your Balance (yes, you can)
We can lower our risk of falling is by practicing balance skill building. Balance ability declines with age (that means from age 35 on). Improving your balance goes hand in hand with strengthening your lower body.

General Balance Tips:
- Focus on a spot straight in front of you instead of the ground.

- Maintain good posture by keeping your chest lifted, your shoulders relaxed, your abdominal muscles braced. And remember to breathe.
- If an exercise is too challenging, hold onto a chair or counter for support until you build confidence.

A Couple of Balance Exercises

Heel-Toe Walk
1. Place the heel of one foot in front of the toes of the other foot. Your forward heel and back toes should touch.
2. Look forward. Focusing on a spot in front of you keeps you steady.
3. Take a step: place the heel directly in front of the toe of your other foot. (Did I say don't look down?)
4. Walk across a room; turn and repeat.

Toe Tap
1. Stand with both feet facing forward.
2. Balance on one leg.
3. Slowly tap the raised toe forward, to the side, to the back and back together.
4. Focus your sight ahead of you, not at the floor.
5. Breathe in and out as you move.
6. Repeat with the other leg

Stretching and Flexibility
As we get older, joints can get stiff and harder to move, limiting their range of motion. When you don't have full

range of motion in a joint, you make smaller movements, setting yourself up for injury.

Why Stretching is so Important
When we are young, we have natural mobility and balance. As we grow older, we lose flexibility. When we're less flexible, we ach more and increase our injury risk. Women are usually more flexible than men, we all lose flexibility. In reality, it is often a matter of inactivity rather than the aging process.

Daily Stretching
At some point, back pain affects an estimated 80% of us. A stretching routine can reduce back stiffness and improve range of motion. Take some time to introduce stretching into your daily regime. It will prevent future injuries and resist ravages that time inflicts on the body.

We can increase our flexibility by stretching and moving every joint in our bodies a few times a week. These three joints, **shoulders**, **knees** and **ankles**, are used every time we reach for something or take a step. These easy exercises can add a spring in our step and reduce pain.

Shoulders:
Our shoulders are the most mobile and complicated joints of our body. If we don't move them, the tissues and muscles shoulder will become stiff.
 1. Stand with your arms at your sides.

2. Raise your arms above your head, bring them back to your shoulder, and lower them back down.

Lower Back:

1. Inhale and reach your right arm up and over your head, slowly bending to the left, with your left arm hanging by your side.
2. Take five deep breaths and return to standing.
3. Repeat on the other side.

Ankles:

1. Ankle stretching improves mobility and pays off in injury prevention.
2. Seated in a chair, extend your leg at the knee and rotate your ankle outward.
3. Pause and then rotate it inward.
4. Repeat with other foot.

Other activities can also be used for flexibility and balance. Some are formal, like yoga. Others may be part of your day, like climbing stairs (hold onto the stair rail. Look where you are going, not at your feet.).

Chapter 4
Step 4: Mood Modifiers — Choose to be Happier

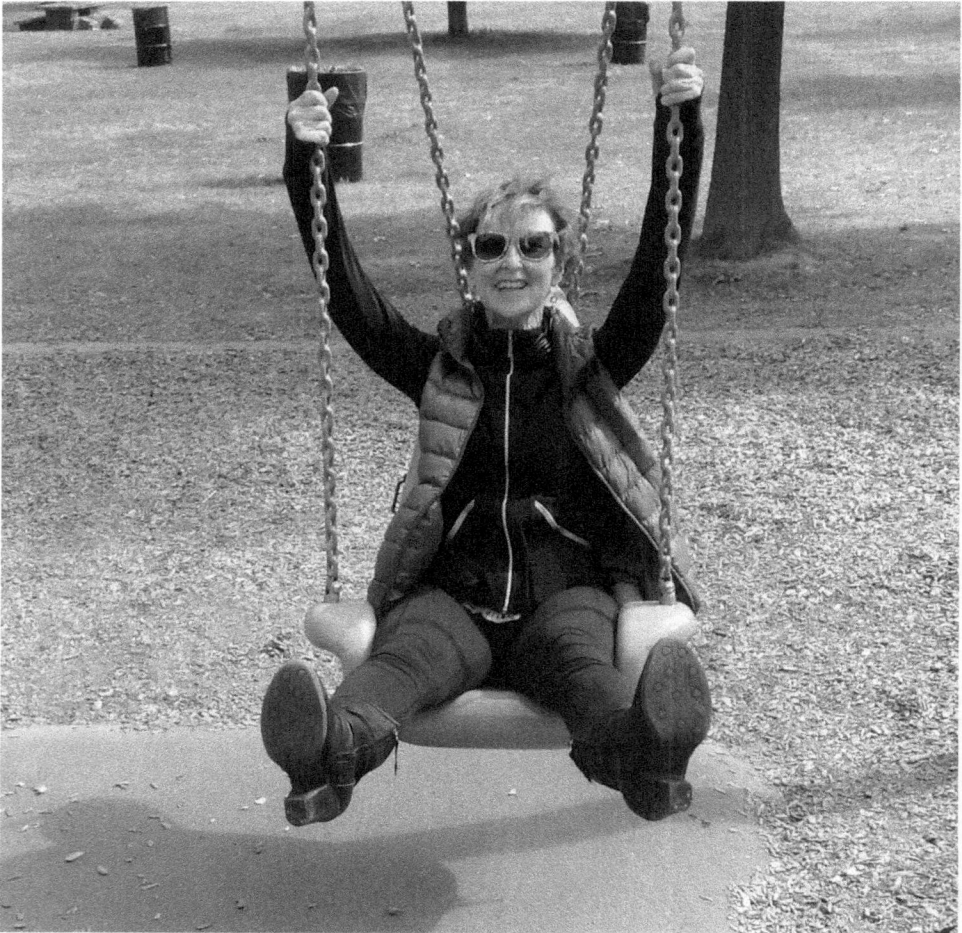

According to Shawn Achor, author of The Happiness Advantage, pursuing happiness leads, not only to happiness, but also to success. Cultivating a positive mindset can boost well-being and improve creativity.

People who cultivate a positive mind-set perform better in the face of challenges.

Happiness Strategy #1: Choose Happy
Happiness depends on how we manage our emotions. Start with a conscious choice to boost your happiness. Many people don't realize that happiness is a choice.

Once we decide to be happier, we can choose strategies to get to a happier state of mind.
- The ability to laugh even as we cry.
- Courage to admit when we're scared
- Confidence to ask for help when we need it
- Nerve to speak up, even if our voice shakes

Many of us give up because we look at how far we have to go, instead of how far we have come. But, although we think we act because of the way we feel, in fact, we often feel because of the way we act. A great attitude always leads to great experiences.

In an "aha" moment, I realized that believing the worst of myself held me back. It prevented me from recognizing and accepting compliments. When I challenged that belief, I became able to change.

Happiness Strategy #2: Cultivate Gratitude
Gratitude can be a tricky thing. There are times when we want what we don't, or cannot, have. Other times we are

so down on ourselves that we cannot even fathom being grateful.

Wherever we go, whatever we do, we can find something to complain about. If we travel, we can complain about lumpy beds and crowded airports. But if we stay home, we can complain that we never go anywhere interesting. Or there's never anything good on television.

So how do we go from a complaining life to one that cultivates a grateful spirit? Try this simple gratitude challenge for 30 days:
    1) Write down 3 things you are grateful for,
    2) Meditate for 2 minutes and
    3) Praise someone.

That's it. I took this challenge. And I can tell you, it will successfully change your attitude.

Happiness Strategy #3: Counteract Negative Thoughts and Feelings

Bad things happen to us every day, some worse than others. Everyone has a choice about how to react to annoyances. You can let them keep you down, or you can move forward. We choose our mood; we choose our happiness. Whether we are in a bad mood or a good mood, we chose that for ourselves. Making a conscious decision to be happy can make us happy.

The key is to make a commitment to do something for ourselves. Here is a truth: *the more we think about something, positive or negative, the more it becomes real.*

Label your thought: Begin to catch yourself as you have a negative thought. When you do, say to yourself, "Hmm, I am experiencing a negative thought." Then remind yourself, "I am only having a thought, not a life sentence." The reminder will help you get rid of negative thoughts. Negativity only has power over you if you react to it.

Replace the negative thought: Using a replacement technique, you replace the thought the moment you recognize it, with a different thought. Without arguing, analyzing, or defending yourself, you cut it off. Instead, immediately replace it with a different thought.

Of course, the key is "*as soon as you recognize it.*" With practice you'll recognize those thoughts sooner and change the thought more quickly.

Happiness Strategy #4: Cultivate Creativity
Breaking into a creative way of life can seem impossible. Watching TV is a common leisure time activity. But it produces some of the lowest levels of happiness. It's the least creative activity we can choose to engage in.

A lot of us believe we don't have a creative bone in our bodies. One of the biggest myths about creativity is that it's bestowed on a lucky few. The reason is that most people see creativity as a luxury. But repositioning creativity into an everyday activity, like breathing, can make it automatic.

Concentrated effort inhibits creativity. And solving creative problems involves considering a lot of options. In fact, focus can keep the creative part of your brain from making associations to solve puzzles. So what, can you do to encourage creative insights?

Relaxing can help our creative juices flow. Relaxation activates our alpha brain wave, so called waves come about when we sit still, with our eyes closed. So, to increase creativity, let yourself stop trying to solve a problem. For example, distract yourself by taking a shower, or going for a walk.

Happiness Strategy #5: Minimize Drama
Minimize drama is my mantra. There is always someone around us to make us feel like there is a crisis going on. That the last thing we can afford right now is to sit still and do nothing. Resist that feeling of always being in crisis mode. Most of the time there is no crisis.

Change your perspective:
1. Pull your conscious focus into the moment. Look at something in front of you (a chair, a plant).
2. Tell yourself right now is the only moment you must focus on.

3. Make decisions as they face you. Facing only the moment is more empowering than putting yourself through the ringer with imagined possibilities.
4. Take three deep breaths and focus on right now. You will notice something called inner peace.

It may take a lot of conscious effort to continuously focus on the moment. After some time, you will notice that you are present and available for yourself more often.

Chapter 5
Step 5: Habit and Rituals — Finding Magic in the Mundane

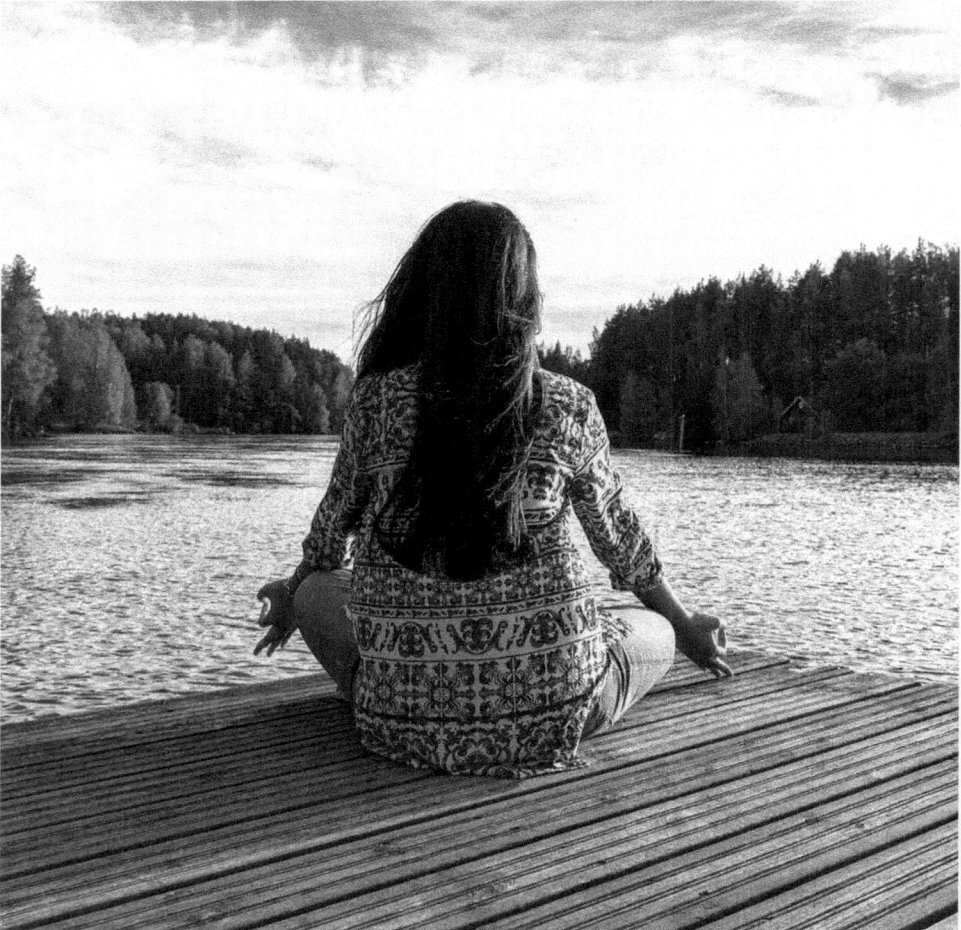

Although often used interchangeably, habit and ritual mean different things. But choose the term that most resonates with you. Consider the differences:

Habit: Desired or not, habits start as something we do. We may intentionally practice an activity. Or we may inadvertently perform an activity repeatedly. After a time, they become a mindless, predictable part of our life; activities like breathing air. A habit, like checking Facebook daily, or brushing our teeth, can be good, bad or indifferent.

Ritual, or routine: We perform rituals with awareness. Bigger than a habit, a ritual supports our flow through life. A practice, ritual, or routine is something positive we choose to do. It focuses on an outcome that enriches our lives and makes us better people. A ritual might include meditating, writing, or reading. Rituals require work and attention. They don't contain us, they expand us. The thing that separates these two acts is mindfulness. You can turn any habit into a ritual by being mindful.

What rituals do you have in your life? What rituals do you need to create in your life? You know the stuff that you KNOW you should be doing if you have any hope of being who you KNOW you should be. Right? Start integrating them into your life.

Creating daily rituals can shape who you are. For better or worse, we are who we are because of the activities we practice throughout the day. To transform our lives for the better, we must make new and better habits.

Building a New Habit/Ritual

Another word for motivation is readiness. Are you READY to change? Many people find change unsettling and try to avoid it.

Think about all the daily actions you take. And examine the insignificant decisions you make throughout the day. What if you make small tweaks to these decisions and actions that could help enhance your life? You make something possible if you are willing to adopt some new empowering rituals.

How Long Will It Take?

Almost everyone has heard that it takes 21 days to form a habit. So, it may be frustrating when you find that you are not getting it. You find, after 21 days, you're only partway to the new behavior you may be working on.

Maxwell Maltz, the doctor credited with establishing the habit timetable, published his thoughts on behavior change, in his book, Psycho-Cybernetics. The book was a blockbuster hit in the 1960s, selling more than 30 million copies. Maltz's work influenced most "self-help" professionals, from Zig Ziglar to Tony Robbins. But everyone forgot that he actually said, "it takes at least 21 days."

That's how society started spreading the myth that it takes 21 days to form a new habit. It's an inviting thought; the time frame is short enough to be inspiring, but long enough to be believable. And who wouldn't like the idea of changing your life in only three weeks?

So, how long does it actually take to form a new habit? And what does all of it mean for you and me?

How Long it Really Takes to Build a New Habit
Phillippa Lally, a health psychology researcher at University College in London, published a study that examined the development of habits of 96 people over a 12-week period. Some people chose simple habits like "drinking a bottle of water with lunch." Others chose more difficult tasks like "running for 15 minutes before dinner."

The results? Lally's study determined that it took anywhere from 18 days to 254 days for people to form a new habit! Developing a new habit varies and depends on behavior and circumstances. She discovered it can take eight months to build a new behavior into your life. So, you want to set realistic expectations.

Reasons why Lally's newer research is inspiring:
1) There is no reason to get down on yourself if something doesn't become a habit after a few weeks. You don't have to judge yourself if you can't master a new behavior in 21 days.
2) Also, it doesn't matter if you mess up every now and then. Making a mistake once or twice has no measurable impact on long-term habits.

3) Understanding the timeline can help us realize that habits are a process. It's hype to think in terms of, "in only 21 Days." Habits never work that way. You have to embrace the process.

Where to Go from Here

At the end of the day, it doesn't matter how long it takes to form a particular habit. you have to put in the work, whether it takes 50 or 500 days. So forget about the number and focus on doing the work.

Small Milestones

Milestones increase focus by reducing the urgency of the project ahead of you. We shouldn't let our goals overwhelm us. Because if they are insurmountable, our journey becomes miserable and discouraging.

If we focus ONLY on our next small milestone goal, we'll feel empowered and motivated.

Don't Beat Yourself Up

We are all human. *Every time we fail, we are one step closer to success.* We have days when we don't feel like doing anything healthy. EVERYONE goes through the same thing, whether in weight loss or any other area of their life! The solution? Start doing it again. That's how you learn anything. That's how you learned how to walk, run, or ride a bicycle.

Every time we fail, we are one step closer to success.

Enjoying what we do, whether it is what we eat or how we are active, is part of what keeps us motivated. Choosing the activities you like will also keep you motivated. You don't get anywhere by beating yourself up. You get there by being kind to yourself, having fun, and learning along the way.

Daily Rituals:
These are things we consistently do on a daily basis that shape the direction of our life, for better or worse.

Morning Rituals:
A morning routine can get our day started productively. Adopt a variety of rituals to build confidence, motivate and create daily momentum.

Evening Rituals:
Empowering evening rituals help us grow. Evenings present us with a perfect opportunity to learn from the day's experiences and lay a path for the next day.

Our habits and rituals are responsible for our successes and our failures. Developing good habits and rituals is more important than self-control in meeting goals.
   Tip #1: Instead of trying to "force" a tough habit into your life all at once, try tackling it in small chunks.
   Tip #2: Maintain accountability by writing it down.
   Tip #3: Focus on positive reinforcement. Self-punishment doesn't reinforce goals. Small rewards

and positive reinforcement are critical for long-term habit change.

Here's some more good news: We can default to positive habits, such as eating a healthy breakfast or going to the gym. Or we can sabotage ourselves. Either is an option.

Building a new habit can be hard if we don't know what our goals are. Pay attention to all the things that you wish were different about yourself. Whatever they may be, those are the habits to develop change.

Keep focused

Once you figure out habits you want, take your first step to get started — focus. Focusing is important to developing habits leading to a happier, more fulfilling, life.

Building Self-discipline

During the process of mastering new habits, it may become difficult. As with everything in life, there are peaks and valleys. There will be days we don't want to get out of bed. And there are other days where we feel great about our progress.

A Chance to Grow

The thing more important than anything else: **enjoy the habit you create**. What kind of life is it if we force ourselves to do things we hate?

The Bottom Line

If you start to make a habit of something you don't like doing, you're almost sure to fail. After a week or two, you'll run out of energy.

In the opposite scenario, i.e., we do something we love doing. Well, how hard is that to motivate ourselves? We look forward to it. When we actually do the habit, our experience is positive and we're happy. That's a habit that is much more likely to stick.

In the end, we have to find something good about a habit to get us going. Successful habit-building means doing what will make us happy on a regular basis.

Here are 3 popular habits many people choose to develop:

MOVE (Exercise) MORE
It's easy to understand why. Exercise plays a role in both physical and mental aspects of our well-being. Most of us hold it as a habit worth pursuing.

There's only one problem… developing an exercise habit a hard habit to form and it takes time to stick. Exercising is harder compared to drinking a glass of water every morning. In fact, it takes at least 66 days to form a regular exercise habit.

How to form an exercise habit
To see lasting results in exercising, increasing our motivation is important. The best way to make exercise a

habit is to start by making a decision that is so easy we can't say no. Here are three strategies you can use in the beginning:

Strategy #1: Most important and one that many people ignore with disastrous results. Choose an activity you enjoy doing. Didn't I say it's hard to form a habit doing something you don't like to do?

Do you hate walking/running on a treadmill? Why would you force yourself to spend a half hour on it? What are the odds of your keeping it up? Spend some time thinking about an activity you'd look forward to doing. Something to give you the fitness benefits you want. Some ideas: running outside, power walking, Zumba, spin class, aqua aerobics.

Strategy #2: Find a way to get started in 2 minutes rather than worrying about your entire workout. Looking for motivation to go for a run? Fill up your water bottle and put on your running shoes. That's all you have to do to consider today's workout a success.

Often, a 2-minute start will be enough to get your motivation flowing get you moving. And if it doesn't, you will have succeeded for 2 minutes. In the big picture, succeeding in the short term is a big deal.

Strategy #3: Set an intention to exercise by filling out this sentence: "During the next week, I will exercise on [DAY] at [TIME OF DAY] at/in [PLACE]."

People who filled out that sentence were 2 to 3 times more likely to exercise over the long run. Taking a formal action is a psychology concept called "implementation intention."

- Find a prompt that gets your brain thinking about the habit you want to develop.
- Choose something to motivate you.
- Actually do the routine.

Once you build the habit of exercise, you can find thousands of ways to improve. Without the habit, every strategy is useless. So, build the habit first, worry about the results later.

SLEEP MORE/SLEEP BETTER
The tough thing about developing a sleep habit is that there is a lot of misinformation, such as the 8-hour rule. There isn't any evidence requiring you to sleep 8 hours a night. It does seem that people who sleep between 6 1/2 and 7 1/2 hours in a night, live the longest, are happier, and more productive. Additionally, you need 5 1/2 hours of sleep for REM (the healing process) to kick in.

Consistency is important. Maintaining regular sleep times reinforces quality sleep.

How to form a habit of better sleep

Our body has an internal clock and hormones that control sleepiness and wakefulness. Our internal clock works best if there is a regular sleep routine. When our internal clock is working well, we feel sleepy at bedtime. We have a window of opportunity for sleep. Going to bed too early can also disturb our sleep.

Exercise in the afternoon can help deepen the sleep experience and reduce the time it takes to fall into dreamland. Make sure to not exercise too late because that can have the reverse effect.

An hour before going to bed, create a relaxing sleep routine. It might include taking a warm bath, reading quietly, or a warm drink. Going to the toilet is also important to avoid having to get up in the middle of the night. Reduce computer and TV screen time near bedtime. Unwind with some form of entertainment that doesn't involve lights and pixels.

EAT BREAKFAST

Eating breakfast ranks high on many of our habit lists. And we often feel guilty if we don't eat breakfast. But don't beat yourself up about breakfast; like all habits, it will take time.

We aren't much better off if we eat something sugary in the morning instead of nothing. Our brain works best with about 25 grams of glucose circulating in the blood stream. That's about the amount found in a banana.

How to form a breakfast habit

Set a realistic goal. If you are not eating breakfast now, it is unrealistic to think you will eat it every day from the start. Think about your weekly lifestyle. Start with one or two days a week to start.

If you're busy or rushed in the morning, prepare as much as possible the night before. Try a small glass of unsweetened fruit juice, a banana, yogurt, or slice of toast. Choose foods you enjoy and ease slowly into the habit eating breakfast.

Chapter 6
Maintenance and Beyond

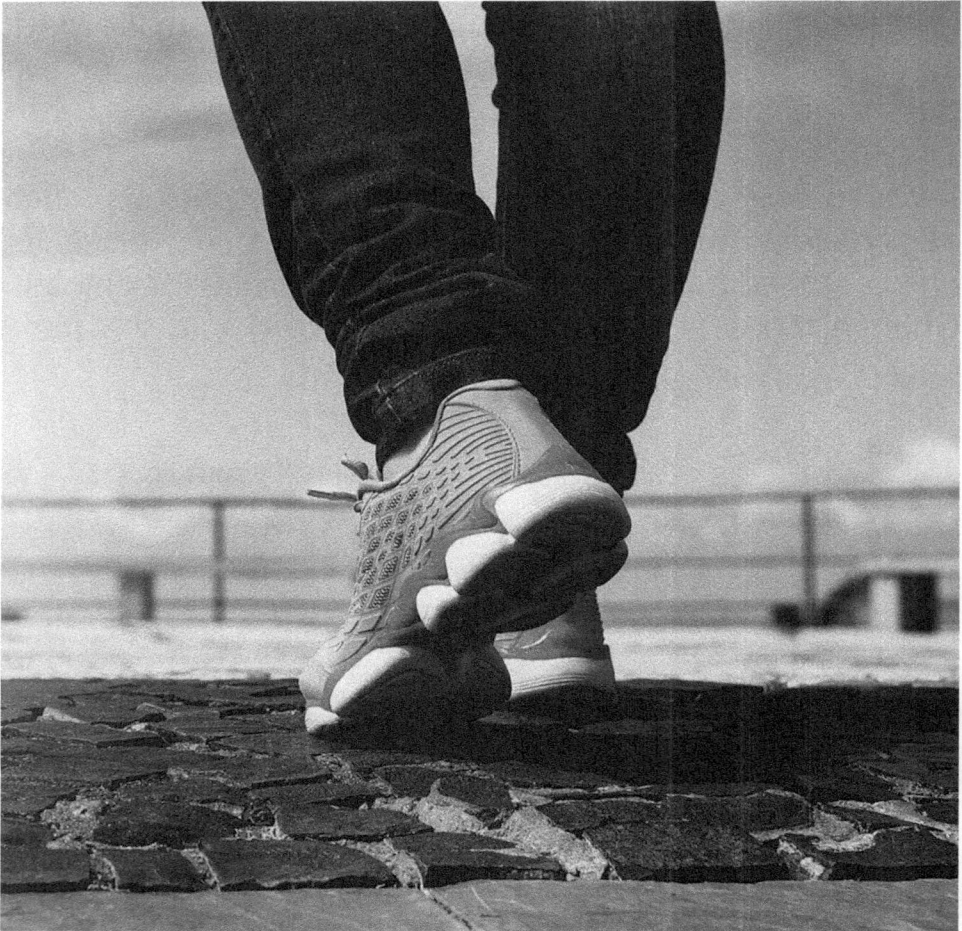

We seldom move through the stages of change in a straightforward, linear path. Instead, we go back and forward before resuming progress. Most of us make several attempts before we change a behavior. Four out of five of us experience some degree of backsliding.

If you experience a lapse or a relapse (a return to old habits) don't give up. Relapsing can be disheartening, but it is not the same as failure. Failure means stopping before we reach our goal. Failure. means never changing our behavior.

Remember, **every time we fail, we are one step closer to succeeding**. So, plan for setbacks, and you can avoid guilt and self-blame. Planning helps us get back on track.

Follow these steps if you have a setback

1. **Forgive yourself.** A setback isn't the end of the world. But abandoning your efforts may make you feel like you are a failure. And you don't have to be.
2. **Give yourself credit for the progress you already made.** You can use your success as motivation to continue. It's important to acknowledge your efforts.
3. **Move on.** To learn from a lapse, use the knowledge to deal with potential setbacks in the future.

Be Patient
Behavior change is like any challenges we encounter at school, at work, or in life in general. It requires us to develop specific skills. We won't master everything in our behavior change program.

View obstacles as challenges that are within your ability to manage. You can tolerate misses and lapses. You can remain motivated. Your behavior change program is an opportunity for personal growth and improvement.

Wellness is the ability to live life with vitality and meaning. Wellness is dynamic and multidimensional. It incorporates physical, emotional, intellectual, spiritual, interpersonal, and environmental dimensions. We can increase motivation by identifying barriers to change.

Commitment is necessary to succeed with a behavior change program. Develop a manageable plan. Arrange social support and stress-management techniques. Track your progress, revising the plan as necessary.

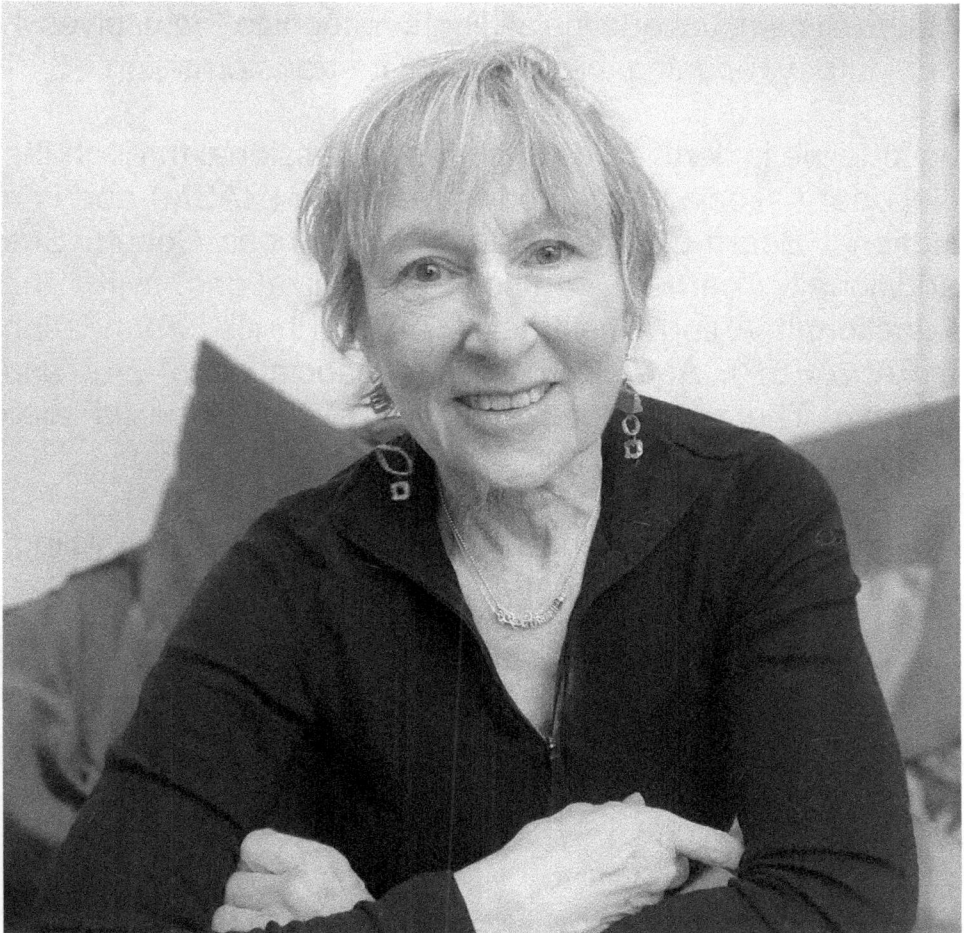

Movement coach and rehab specialist, health & wellness coach, Jacqueline Gikow is the owner of Audacious Living NYC, specializing in pain relief through better movement. She supports your determination to hurt less, grow stronger, and prevent reinjury.

Jacqueline maintains a holistic professional practice of health and wellness. From managing pain from her own injuries and health challenges, she became empathetic to others in pain. Jacqueline's clients recognize themselves in her journey, opening the possibility for transformation.

Jacqueline is certified as a fitness professional through the National Association of Sports Medicine (NASM) and is a National Board-Certified Health & Wellness Coach. She additionally carries certified specializations with the Functional Aging Institute (FAI), Arthritis Foundation (AFAP/AFEP), Aquatic Exercise Association (AEA), and Aquatic Therapy Rehab Institute (ATRI). She is also certified as an arthritis program leader.

An unabashed techie and DIY nerd, Gikow loves bicycling, bright colors, cats, and hats.

$59 Special Offer

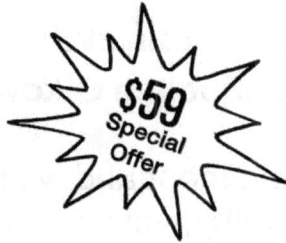

A special offer, to readers of my book
Special offer $59* includes: 3 30-minute remote sessions

Why work with me?
A book offers information to reach a wide audience. These 3 introductory, one-on-one online sessions provide personalized workout guidance:
• Adjust form to ensure effective movement •
• Assess movement quality for safety •
• Explore specific exercises for individual goals •

*Regular individual 30-minute remote session fee: $60

Audacious**L**ivingNYC™
Jacqueline Gikow

Personalized movement and wellness coaching.
Get started on a healthy, active and vital life, now and tomorrow.

Email: jacquelinegikow@gmail.com
Phone: 917.301.3952

Website: https://audaciouslivingnyc.com
Instagram, Twitter & YouTube: @JacquelineGikow

www.ingramcontent.com/pod-product-compliance
Lightning Source LLC
Chambersburg PA
CBHW071342290326
41933CB00040B/2087